When Someone You Love Has Cancer

A Guide to Help Kids Cope

Written by
Alaric Lewis, OSB

Illustrated by
R. W. Alley

D0817304

To The Leaf

Text © 2005 Alaric Lewis, OSB
Illustrations © 2005 St. Meinrad Archabbey
Published by One Caring Place
Abbey Press
St. Meinrad, Indiana 47577

Library of Congress Catalog Number
2005905616

ISBN 0-87029-395-8

Printed in the United States of America

A Message to Parents, Teachers, and Other Caring Adults

Few things affect the everyday life of a family like the presence of a lingering illness like cancer. Surgeries, chemotherapy, radiation, check-ups, relapses not only take a toll on one's time, but they sap energies, heighten worries, promote fears, and bring despair. Coping with the situations arising from cancer is an arduous task—not only for the one suffering illness, but for the entire family.

These struggles can be amplified for children. While adults have the ability to better understand the complexities of cancer, and the responsibilities to keep the family going, children experience much confusion, fear, and misunderstanding about the disease and its treatment. Frequently, children are lost in the shuffle of it all, wandering and wondering what is happening, and what their role is. Although naturally resilient, children are not immune to the same pressures experienced by adults.

Adults need to remember that children's responses and needs are different from their own. When I was a young boy and my mother was dying of Hodgkin's Disease, many caring adults wanted to "spare" me from the grim realities of her illness, feeling that I was too young to understand. Yet, the questions I had about the events that swirled around my world were very real. Given the lack of real answers, I frequently resorted to my own misinformed hypotheses. Children are never too young to understand some sort of explanation, and adults need to remember that talking with the child is vital for his or her understanding, self-awareness, and eventual ability to cope.

Faced with such confusion, a child may act out, becoming petulant or irritable. Patience—frequently in short supply during difficult times—needs to rule the day. Making sure the child has time to be a child, enjoying fun and play, and entering into that play time with the child, will help temper these actions.

May this book help children cope with the presence of cancer in their lives. May it guide them to a healthier understanding of how the disease affects their loved one, their family, and their world. May it offer—as much as is possible—a little healing in the midst of sickness.

—Alaric Lewis, OSB

What Is Cancer?

Your body is like a machine, made up of many parts that make up bigger parts, that make up still bigger parts. The smallest part is called a *cell*, and a cell is so small you can't even see it with your eyes—you would need a microscope. But cells grouped together make *tissues*. And tissues working together make *organs*. And organs make us able to breathe and eat and pump blood and fight against sickness.

Sometimes something bad happens to the cells, and these sick cells group together. When they do, it can cause harm to tissues and organs in the body, making a person sick. This is called *cancer*.

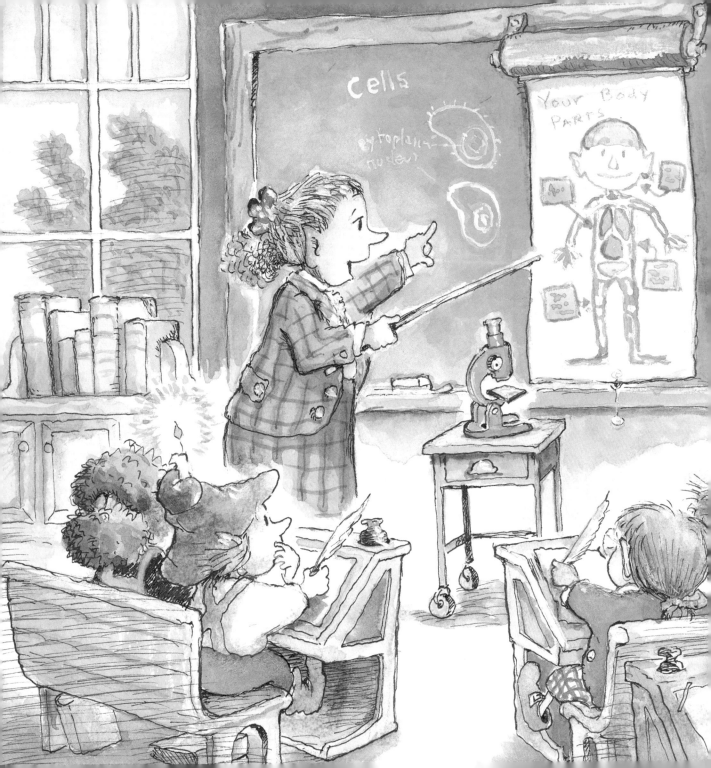

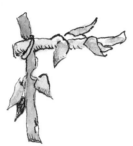

Don't Be Afraid to Ask Questions

There are many types of cancer, and each can harm different parts of the body. You might want to know exactly what is happening in the body of someone you love.

Ask a relative or teacher to explain what part of your loved one's body is hurting. They can help you look up things in an encyclopedia or on the Internet. There are pictures and facts there about the tissues or organs harmed by the cancer. They can help you understand the difference between a healthy body (like yours) and a sick one.

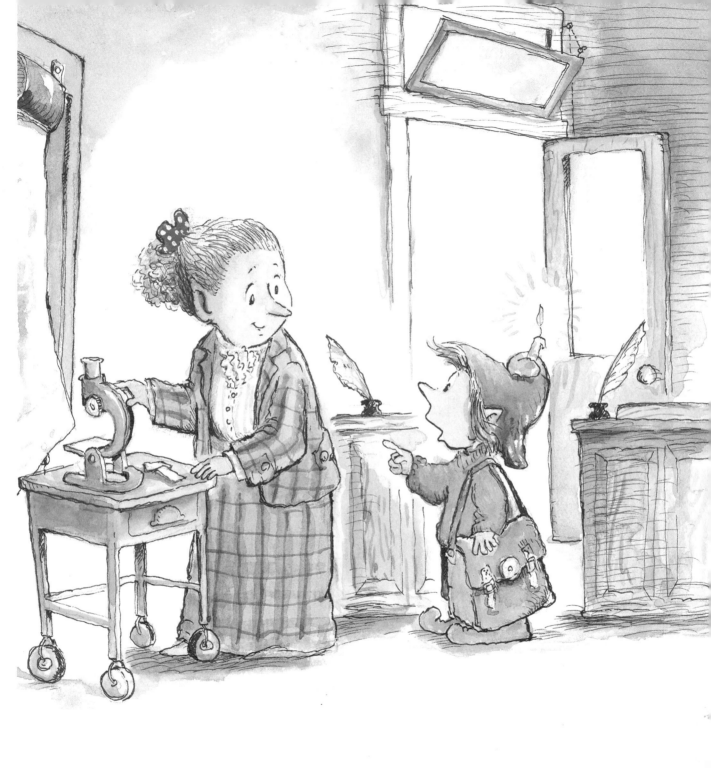

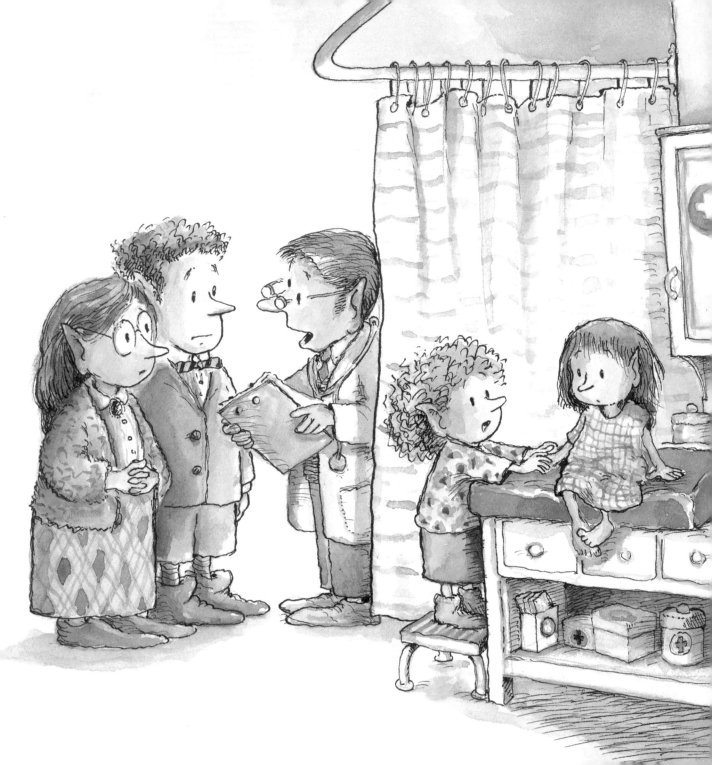

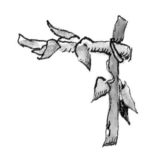

Scary Words Are Not Always So Scary

Sometimes you may hear people say big words that you don't understand. These words can sound very scary, like: *biopsy, chemotherapy, remission*.

Have someone help you understand these words (and any other words you might hear). When you know what they mean, you'll see they're not so scary after all. For example, *biopsy* means "exploring to see what might be wrong." *Chemotherapy* means "cleaning the inside of the body to try and help the sick cells." And *remission* means the best thing of all: "the person is better now."

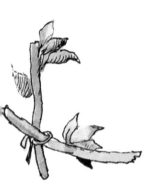

It's Not Your Fault

It's natural to want to know why something happens. You might be wondering why Grandpa Pete has cancer. Doctors know that some things (like smoking cigarettes) can cause cancer. But there is still much they don't know, and they can never answer the "why" for sure.

If we don't know why, sometimes we may wonder if **we** did something to make this happen. We might think no one is telling us "why" because it is somehow our fault.

But people get sick, and that's just the way things are sometimes. Know that you did nothing to bring this on.

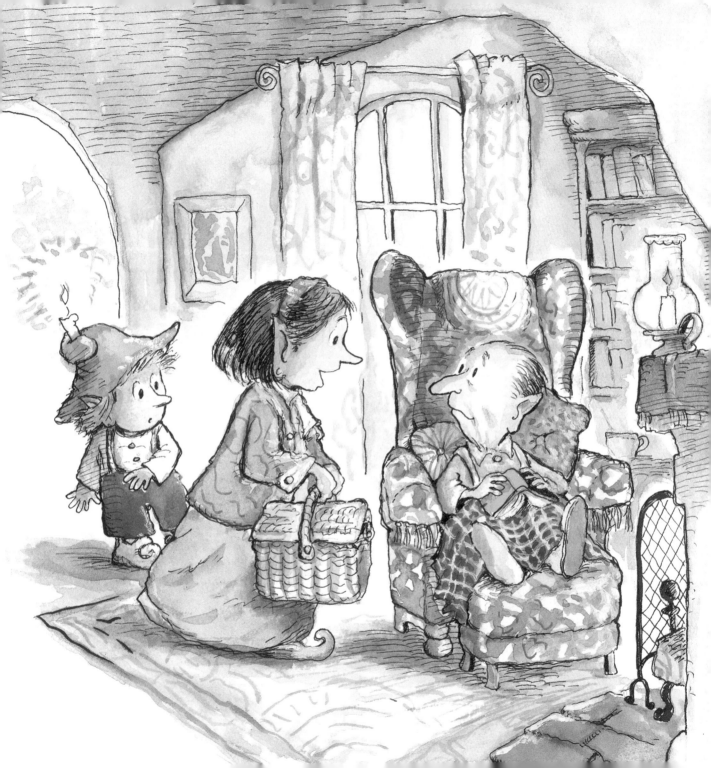

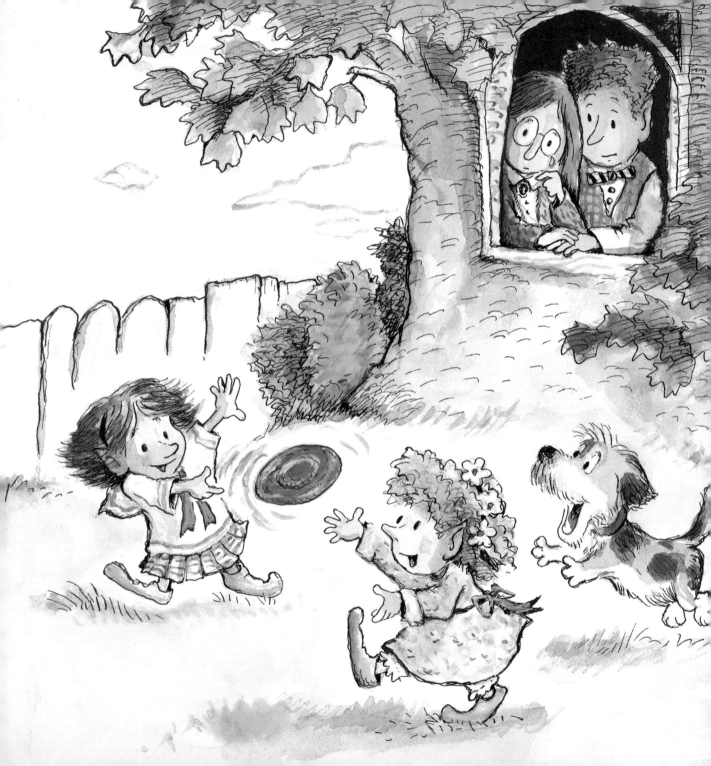

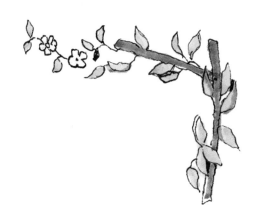

It's OK to Cry

When someone has cancer, it can be very sad for everyone. No one likes to see someone they love hurting. And when you know he or she **is** hurting, it can make **you** hurt also. This causes sadness for everyone: for the person who is sick, for family members, and for you.

It's OK to be sad, and it's OK to cry. Crying doesn't mean you're not strong. It's just a way for your body to show you are sad. Everyone cries: boys and girls, men and women. And it's OK for you, too, if you feel like it.

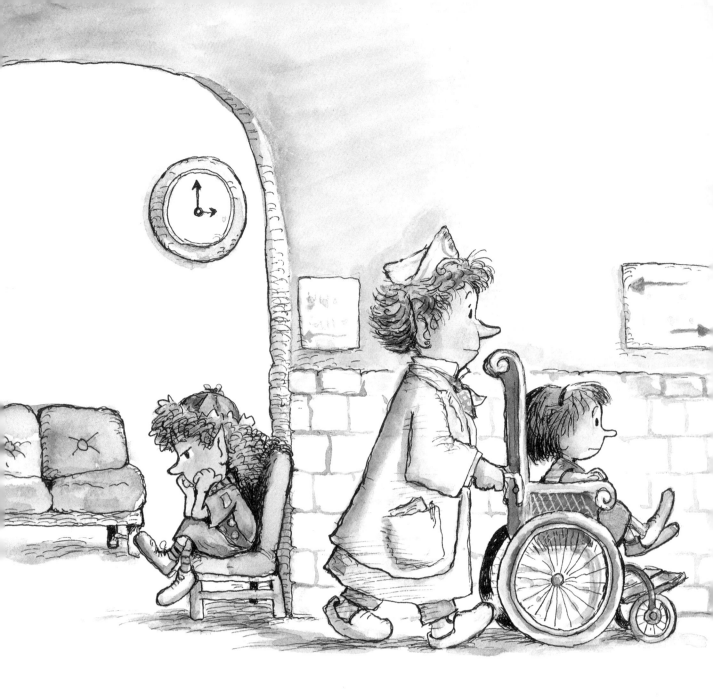

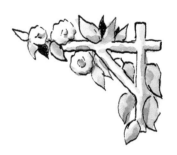

It's OK to Be Mad

When someone in your family has cancer, life can be even busier than usual. Along with all your normal activities like school and soccer and Scouts, time also has to be made for your loved one's needs. There will be extra trips to the hospital for check-ups and chemotherapy. Sometimes, this means that you might not get to do what you like to do. And this could make you mad.

It's OK to be mad, especially when things are hard to understand. When you get to do something fun again, you'll be less mad.

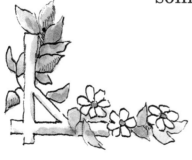

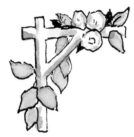

It's OK to Be Afraid

Even if you know something about it, cancer can still be scary. There might be a thousand questions running through your mind, like "What if Bobby doesn't get better?" or, "What if Sarah never comes home from the hospital?" You might wonder if things will ever get back to normal again.

Being afraid doesn't mean you're being a baby. It just means that there are things going on that are hard to understand, and that's scary for everyone—even grown-ups. Remember, you can always tell them that you are afraid.

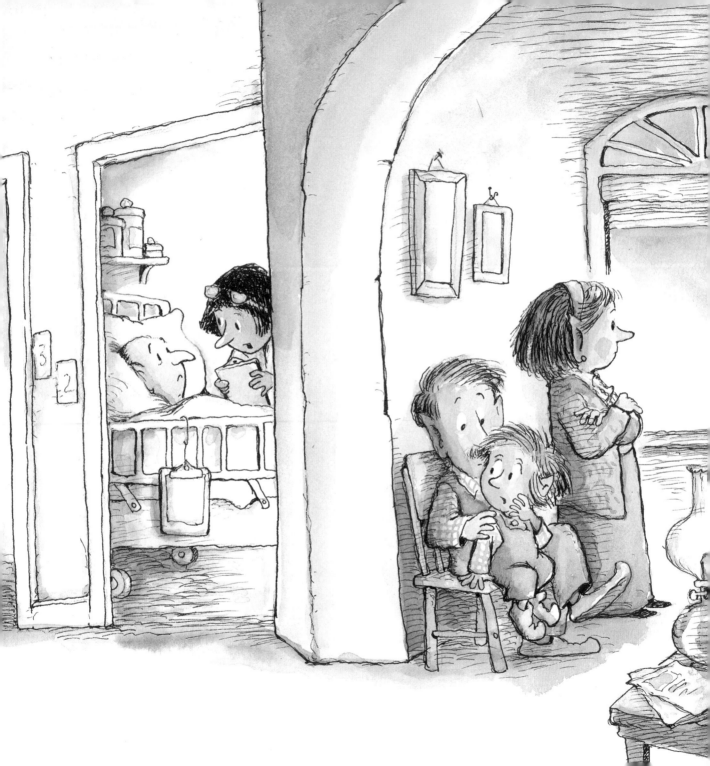

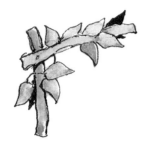

It's OK to Be Happy

There is much to be sad, mad, and afraid about when someone you love has cancer. But there are still things to be happy about, and it's good to remember that, too.

Maybe your dog did something crazy. Maybe you heard a funny story at school. Maybe you scored a goal at your soccer match. When these things happen, don't be afraid to laugh and roll your eyes and be happy. Your loved one who is sick will want to hear about it, too. By sharing happiness with her, she'll be able to smile, too.

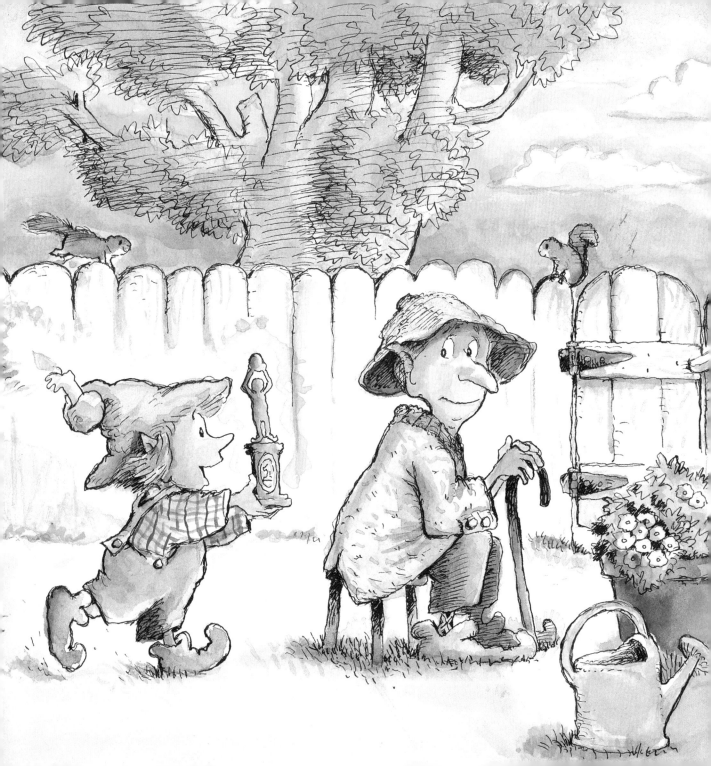

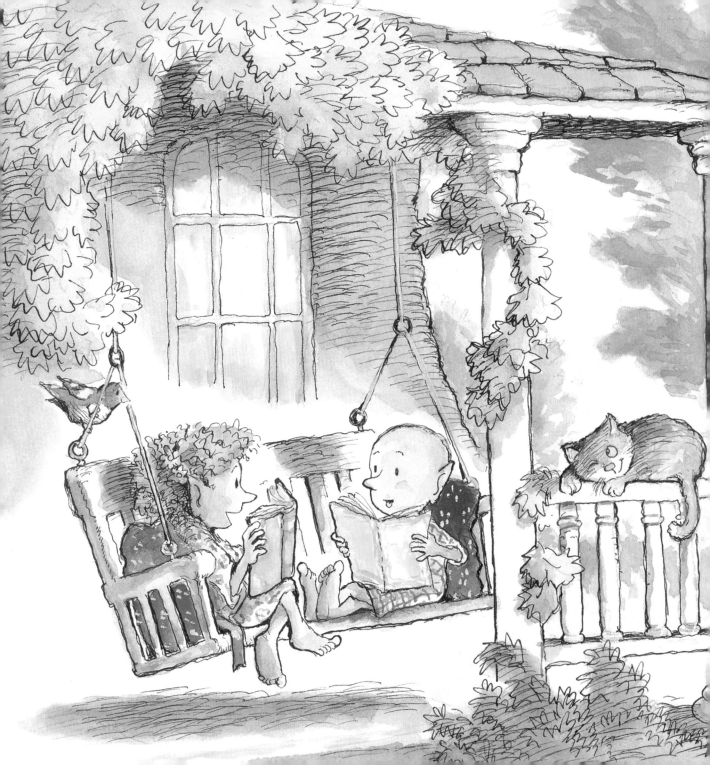

Talking Helps

Sometimes you will feel sad, sometimes mad, sometimes afraid, and sometimes happy. Since everyone is different, you may feel some things that others don't. Your cousin may be happy when you're sad. You may be afraid when your sister is mad.

When there are so many different feelings happening around you, it's good to talk to someone to help understand them all better. If possible, a good person to talk to is the loved one who has cancer. But, there are many people who want to hear how you feel: parents, teachers, ministers, relatives.

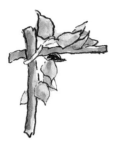

People Change

When someone is fighting against cancer, many things happen that change that person. Your favorite aunt, who always played ball or climbed trees with you, may become tired and unable to do much. Or she may lose weight and become much smaller. Some people who have dark skin may become very pale. Some people lose all of their hair.

What's important is on the *inside* of a person. If you notice changes in Aunt Karen, don't be afraid. It is what her body must go through while she's fighting against the disease. Know that what's inside—the person who loves you—remains the same.

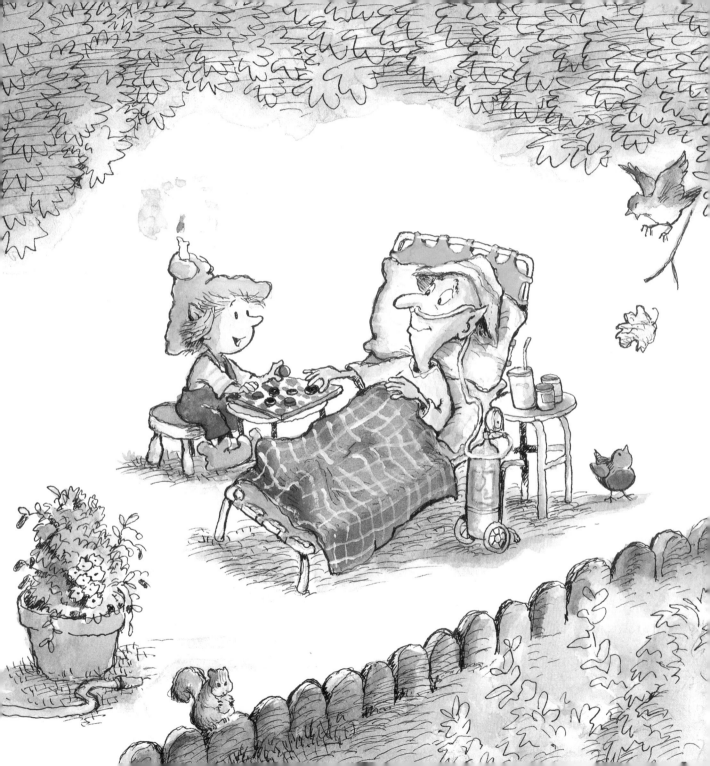

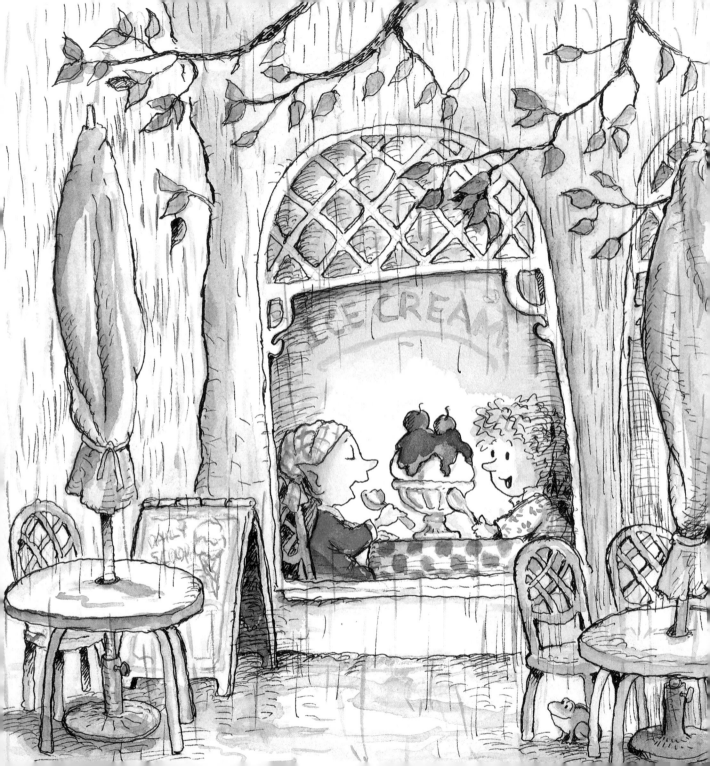

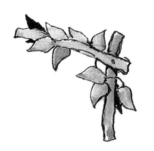

Do Something Nice

Think back to when you had a cold or the flu, or maybe when you got your tonsils out. Being sick is no fun! No one likes to feel bad, and no amount of ice cream can help that. But it helps when people do nice things to show they care.

You can help your loved one feel better by doing something nice for him. Maybe you can make a card with pictures of happy things. Or pick flowers to brighten up his room. Or tell him about something exciting that happened at school.

When you help someone to feel better, you'll find that you feel better, too.

Sometimes People Don't Get Better

Cancer is a very serious disease. Sometimes, even though doctors try very hard and we pray and hope very much, the person we love may not get better. This doesn't mean the doctors didn't do their job, or that our prayers were not answered. It just means the cancer became too strong to fight.

If this happens, you might not be able to visit your loved one as much for a while, because he must spend more time in the hospital. It may even mean that his life here will end, and he will go to heaven.

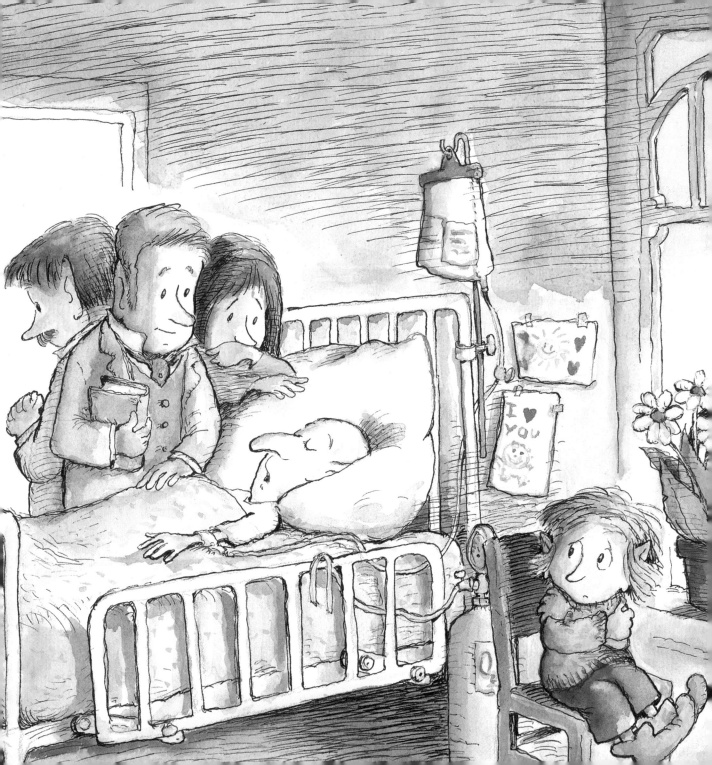

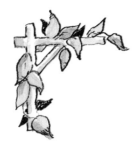

You Will Be Taken Care Of

You may worry about who will care for you if your loved one is not around: Who will fix my breakfast? Who will take me to school? Who will read me stories?

If you are worried about this, talk to a grown-up. You will find there will be many people who will help you—all you need to do is ask. Always remember there are many caring adults who will make sure you have the things you need.

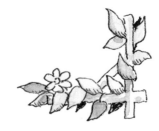

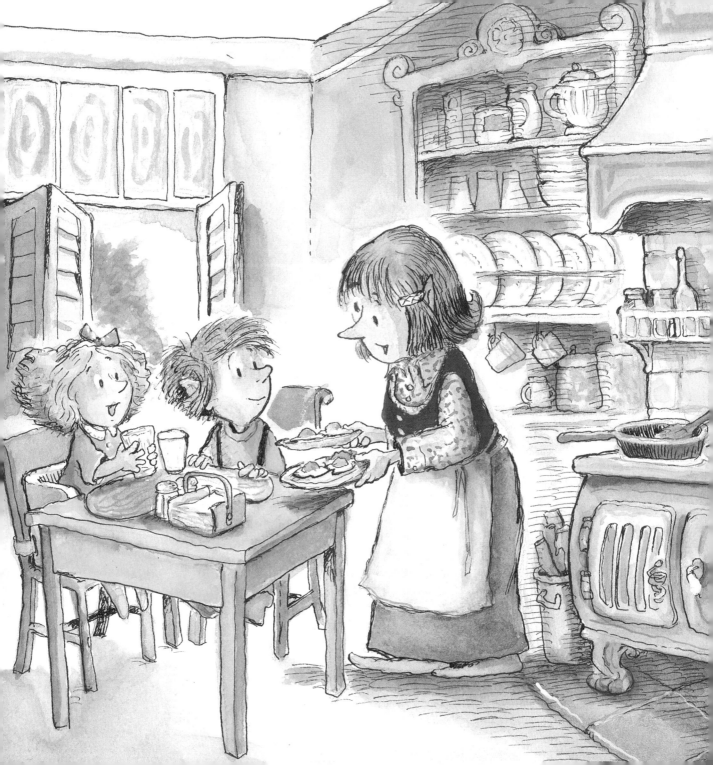

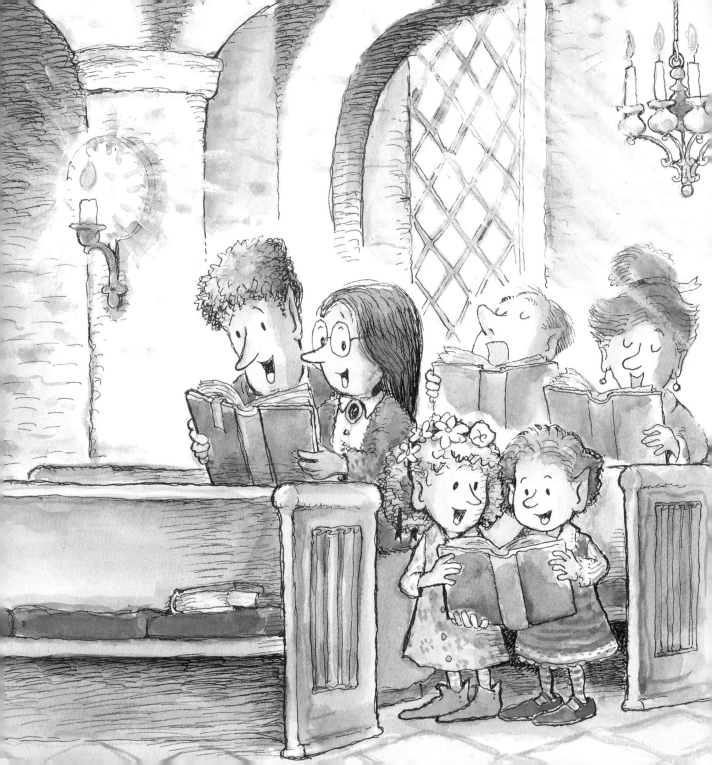

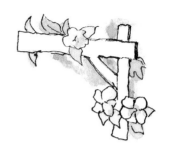

Say a Prayer

Many people pray when they need extra help—especially when someone is sick. Praying is asking God to give us, and the people we love, the things we need most.

You can pray for your loved one as well. Ask a grown-up, like a priest or minister, or even your parents, to help you pray so that your loved one may get the things she needs most.

God listens to all prayer, so you can pray in your own way. You can ask God to help your loved one, and say a prayer of thanks when your loved one is feeling better.

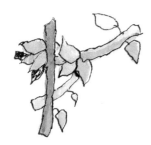

Alaric Lewis, OSB, is a monk of Saint Meinrad Archabbey, a community of Benedictines located in southern Indiana. A Catholic priest, Father Alaric is a popular retreat master and writer with extensive experience in the parish. Father Alaric, himself, is a cancer survivor. In addition to losing his mother to cancer when he was a child, his sister is also a cancer survivor. Currently involved in doctoral studies in Rome, he has also served as associate editor for the Abbey Press publications division, One Caring Place. He is the author of the books *A Healing Year: Daily Meditations for Living with Loss, PrayerStarters in Times of Pain or Illness,* and *Music Therapy*; he has also written the CareNotes *Living as a Cancer Survivor* and *Five Ways to Help Someone Living with Cancer*.

R. W. Alley is the illustrator for the popular Abbey Press adult series of Elf-help books, as well as an illustrator and writer of children's books. He lives in Barrington, Rhode Island, with his wife, daughter, and son.